"Bruce Stein has written an excellent and very readable 'user's manual' for Positive Airway Pressure therapy devices (CPAP/BiPAP). I put user's manual in quotations because, as the author reminds the reader regularly, his book does not replace the instructions provided by the manufacturer.

"Mr. Stein addresses a number of the issues that can interfere with the successful use of therapy. One example is using the device while traveling. He provides a checklist of items traveling apneics should have on hand to address any eventuality.

"For those new to therapy, this book should go a long way to flattening the learning curve tto successfully treating your condition." — **Ed Grandi, Executive Director, American Sleep Apnea Association, Washington, DC**

"I think it [this book] will be a big help to users, especially those who lack Bruce's ingenuity. I plan to read it again." — **Mike Glenn, Galesburg, MI**

"I've used a CPAP for 15 years. If it takes a while to get used to it, don't give up. You're not only extending your own life but giving your spouse an opportunity to get some decent rest as well. This well written book will help you use your unit easier." — **Lowell Seyburn, Portage, MI**

"Excellent. I have used CPAP for almost two decades and I learned a number of useful things. I would strongly recommend for anyone diagnosed with sleep apnea and prescribed CPAP or BiPAP." — **Paul Nimz, Vicksburg, MI**

". . . It encourages users to stick with the device by citing some of the severe health risks associated with not taking sleep apnea seriously. My husband never uses his unit when we travel because of some of the very concerns that Bruce addresses. If I have to, I will read this book aloud to [him . . . to] acquire suggestions on how to tweak his system to fit his needs." — **Vera Tiani, Plymouth, IN**

Sleep Apnea and CPAP

Sleep Apnea and CPAP:
A User's Manual By A User

How to Use CPAP or BiPAP
Easily
or
How I Overcame Problems With
CPAP

by Bruce Stein

Revised Edition

Kalamazoo Publishing
Kalamazoo, Michigan

Kalamazoo Publishing
Kalamazoo, Michigan, USA, 49009
www.kazoopub.com

*ISBN 978-0-9831991-2-0

Stein, Bruce
    Sleep apnea and CPAP: a user's
manual by a user. Revised ed. Kalamazoo,
Mich.: Kalamazoo Publishing, 2011.
    xxxii, 91p. Includes index
    1. Sleep apnea syndrome—Treatment
2. Sleep disorders—Treatment 3. Respira-
tion—Apparatus, equipment, materials I.
Title
616.8498 S818 rev

DEDICATION

This book is dedicated to my late father, Sam I. Stein, PhD, MD, who had sleep apnea that directly contributed to his death in 1969 at age 62.

As a young child, I remember lying in bed hearing my dad *snore.* You might ask, "If you were a young child, you should have been asleep long before your parents went to bed. If you were in bed asleep, how could you hear your dad snoring?" Good question.

Simple answer. His snoring was such that he woke the neighbors for a two blocks radius. At the time, I did not know that the gasping I heard with his every breath was sleep apnea. The decreased oxygen to his heart muscle probably was a significant contributing factor to his fatal heart attack.

CONTENTS

LIST OF PICTURES

~

PREFACE

Overcoming Common Problems

This is a User's Manual, not a treatise on sleep apnea or CPAP. It assumes that the reader has been diagnosed with sleep apnea and has been told to use CPAP. However, it does not assume that the reader knows how to operate a CPAP system, including both the machine and mask. In fact, I have found that too many people diagnosed with sleep apnea *don't* know how to use the device, have serious problems with it, and therefore don't use it regularly and ultimately quit using it. That is the reason I wrote this book.

When I was first diagnosed with sleep apnea in November of 1999, I didn't know anything about sleep apnea, CPAP[1] or

---

[1] CPAP refers to Continuous Positive Airway Pressure and BiPAP refers to Bi-level Positive Airway Pressure, meaning two levels of pressure; a higher one for inhale and a lower one for exhale. Whatever is

BiPAP nor did I know anyone that had the condition. However, because I worked at a large pharmaceutical company that employed a few thousand workers, I quickly learned that many of my colleagues used CPAP.

As I listened to their tales of woe, I quickly realized that many had tried to use their CPAP and had given up. Some people used CPAP on some days but not other days; others used it part of the night and then quit sometime during the night for various reasons. Still others used it at home but did not take it when they traveled. And others never used CPAP for various reasons. Having fought with my machine and won the battle, I want to pass along to others the information and tips I have learned that make using CPAP or BiPAP much easier. It is my hope that CPAP users will use it whenever they sleep.

The rationale for not using CPAP ranged from having problems with the equipment

---

said in this book regarding CPAP is equally applicable to BiPAP. Because CPAP is much more common than BiPAP, I will use the term CPAP to refer to both CPAP and BiPAP.

to lack of concern about being tired during the day. Almost no one was concerned about their blood-oxygen levels dropping or having a heart attack.

After I was diagnosed with sleep apnea, I quickly did some research on the importance of treating it. I became aware that it was critically important for someone diagnosed with sleep apnea to always use CPAP so their blood-oxygen levels did not drop. While sleep apnea is a contributing factor to death by heart attacks, such as the situation with my dad, I found out that few users were aware of this important connection.

At that point, I too was having what seemed like insurmountable problems with my BiPAP equipment. In particular:

- For some unknown reason, the literature that came with my first machine said put the machine on the floor, not a table and I found I was having trouble with it at that lower level.

- The biggest problem came when I rolled over. The tube got caught in the bedding, pulled on the mask, twisted it and therefore the seal did not work.

- I was having trouble taking a ring out of the main mask piece since my fingers did not fit in the area. Two very small screw drivers did the job until I learned how to get my fingers inside. In addition, I was having trouble putting the mask together properly at night.

- There were a number of problems when I traveled. Some places did not have a grounded outlet, in others the outlet was too far from the bed, or I could not hang the tube as I did at home, etc.

I quickly understood the problems that others were having and why some abandoned CPAP all together. Rather than run with the crowd, I decided to stay and fight. It became apparent that if I made a number of changes with my BiPAP, things would work better. This User's Manual sets forth what I have learned and the modifications I have made to make BiPAP workable for me.

For a number of years, I have taught a course twice a year in Portage, Michigan, for Continuing Education on Sleep Apnea and CPAP. I have been amazed at what I have learned. Some users only wash their mask occasionally. Others wash it, but never take it apart. Some were unaware that there are coverings for the tubing when the humidifier is used. Many complained that their masks did not fit. Some had no idea how to travel with CPAP; there is an entire chapter devoted to that.

In this User's Manual, I have tried to provide information on how I solved the problems that I have had as well as problems others have encountered so that you will not have to go through all the hassle that I did. I do not want anyone have sleep apnea to contribute to their death as it did to my father's death.

While "Barbara BiPAP" and I did hop into bed the first night, it took time for us to build a relationship to the point that we got along very well. This is a story of how our relationship grew and developed to where we were are a happy couple. Then it became apparent that "Barbara" was aging; there were newer younger sleeker, slimmer models which were more current in the

world (internal humidifier), more fun and much easier to travel with. So after 10 years "Barbara I" and I parted ways.
I quickly picked up with "Barbara II;" we hit it off together right from the start and today we are a happy couple. Hopefully, I can explain some of the things that make us a happy couple to you, so you and your CPAP will have an excellent relationship in the future.

PREFACE to the REVISED EDITION

Many positive comments were received regarding the first publication including suggestions for improvement. These included everything from simple typos to suggestions for rewording to make the subject more understandable.

Importantly, the book was reviewed by a very experienced cardiologist who has sleep apnea, and a vendor of sleep apnea supplies. Both of these reviewers offered a number of helpful suggestions for improvement that have been incorporated into this revision.

In addition, three more pictures have been added showing a slim tube covering, the couplers and a way of using the rubber band system when the bed is not up against a wall and no ceiling hook nor wall support is available. Because at least two of the Internet links in the first version are no longer in use and others may not be in the near future, all Internet links have been replaced by a discussion of the subject matter.

~

IMPORTANT NOTICE

STOP - Warning

This book is how Barbara BiPAP and I met, jumped into bed together the first night, began a rocky and difficult relationship, but worked through our problems. Since I could not change Barbara, to improve our relationship I had to modify how we related.

After a period of trial and error we developed an excellent relationship. During this period of adjustment and afterwards I did not always follow the directions of the manufacturer for use and/or cleaning. This book describes what I have done to get my relationship to work for me; it is not necessarily what you should do. Your equipment may be different than mine and our situations may well be different. To the extent that what I do differs from the directions of the manufacturer of your equipment – you should follow the directions of your manufacturer.

Your CPAP/BiPAP machine, tube and mask come with directions for use and cleaning which have been developed by the manufacturer. I repeat—you should follow the directions of your manufacturer/vendor.

Further, it is best to use your system seven days a week, 365 days a year. But if for some reason you can't, don't give up. It is not all or nothing. Six days a week is better than five days week. The more often you can use it the better for you. But if you can't take it on a trip or can't use it for some other reason, don't feel like a failure. It is much like dieting. There is theoretical perfection and there is reality in practice. I use mine every night because the hassle in doing so is worth the rested feeling in the morning and the knowledge that I am taking care of my body. If the problems outweigh the benefits for a particular circumstance, either accept that or work to reduce the problems so the benefits outweigh them. But just because you can't use it all the time, don't give up.

The Real Dangers of Not Using CPAP for Those Who Have Sleep Apnea

While this is a user manual for those who have been diagnosed with sleep apnea and for whom CPAP has been prescribed, a brief note about (obstructive) sleep apnea is here because, surprisingly, I found many of those who have been diagnosed with sleep apnea and are trying to use CPAP did not have a good understanding of sleep apnea or its dangers.

Obstructive sleep apnea is a sleep disorder characterized by a blockage of the airway, usually when the soft tissue in the rear of the throat closes the airway during sleep. The individual usually becomes aware of the problems because of a high degree of daytime sleepiness and fatigue. Clinically the condition is diagnosed during a sleep study in which the number of apneic events is measured by a polysomnogram. Snoring, while common with those who have sleep apnea is a not a reliable diagnostic indicator.

There are four non-REM (Rapid Eye Movement) stages of sleep that precede REM sleep, which is the restful stage. So an individual needs to go through the other four cycles successfully to get to the fifth and restful stage, REM. During a night one will go through the five stages of sleep as many as five times.

An apneic event occurs when soft tissue of an individual's throat blocks air flow or breathing. This breathing stoppage can occur five to more than 50 times an hour throughout the night. When breathing stops, oxygen de-saturation in the brain begins with a concomitant build-up of carbon dioxide. These conditions force the sleeper to gasp for breath, which is what interrupts sleep. When these constant arousals occur, the individual's normal sleep pattern is interrupted and he/she does not reach REM sleep. The individual, therefore, is not rested in the morning, but rather may feel it is time to go to bed rather than get up.

Even though a person with sleep apnea may sleep for hours, the quality of sleep is poor, which is what causes tiredness the next day. Because of excess daytime sleepiness and/or fatigue there is a danger of falling asleep while driving or having an accident while operating machinery. In addition, sleep apnea is associated with irritability, depression, anxiety, stress, daytime headaches, sexual dysfunction and poor memory.

The second danger occurs when breathing is interrupted. The blood-oxygen concentration in the blood decreases, putting a strain on heart, brain and other tissue. This can lead to high blood pressure, stroke, cardiac arrhythmia and heart attack. Dr. Neomi Shah of Yale University reported in May 2007, in the *Science Daily* on a study of 1,132 patients referred for sleep apnea evaluation. The study showed that sleep apnea, if not treated, over a period of four or five years increases the risk of a heart attack or death by 30 percent.

Researchers at the Mayo Clinic found that individuals with untreated sleep apnea have an increased risk of having a heart attack during the time they sleep (12am to 6am). This research was published in the July 2008 issue of the *Journal of the American College of Cardiology*. According to Dr. Virend Somers, a cardiologist and lead author, a disproportionate share of heart attacks occur between 6am and noon. The study evaluated 92 patients admitted because of a heart attack. Of those with a heart attack between 12am and 6am, 91% had sleep apnea. A word to the wise, if you have sleep apnea and want to decrease your chances of having a heart attack, one very important thing you can do is use your CPAP all the time.

~

SLEEP WISDOM

The importance of getting a good night's sleep is demonstrated not only by the medical literature but also by the amazing number of quotes of nonscientists regarding sleep. These individuals, from all walks of life, all came to the same conclusion as to the critically important requirement of a good night's sleep. Their wisdom should impress upon the reader the necessity of individuals with sleep apnea to use their CPAP regularly.

I believe the greatest asset a head of state can have is the ability to get a good night's sleep.
— Harold Wilson

Laugh and the world laughs with you, snore and you sleep alone.
— Anthony Burgess

Sleep is the best meditation.
— Dalai Lama

Silence is the sleep that nourishes wisdom.
— Francis Bacon

That we are not much sicker and much madder than we are is due exclusively to that most blessed and blessing of all natural graces, sleep.
— Aldous Huxley

It is a common experience that a problem difficult at night is resolved in the morning after the committee of sleep has worked on it.
— John Steinbeck

Sorrow can be alleviated by good sleep, a bath and a glass of wine.
— Thomas Aquinas

The minute anyone's getting anxious I say, you must eat and you must sleep. They're the two vital elements for a healthy life.
— Francesca Annis

Sleep is that golden chain that ties health and our bodies together.
— Thomas Dekker

I think sleep's really important. I value it as much as waking up and having a full day.
— Jena Malone

Think in the morning. Act in the noon. Eat in the evening. Sleep in the night.
— William Blake

It is better to sleep on things beforehand than lie awake about them afterwards.
— Baltasar Gracián

True silence is the rest of the mind, and is to the spirit what sleep is to the body, nourishment and refreshment
— William Penn

There is a time for many words, and there is also a time for sleep.
— Homer

I'm lucky, I can sleep from takeoff until we land; so I'm fresh, rested and ready to work on arrival.
— Eva Herzigova

Man should forget his anger before he lies down to sleep.
— Mohandas Gandhi

I love sleep. My life has the tendency to fall apart when I'm awake, you know?
— Ernest Hemingway

Have courage for the great sorrows of life
and patience for the small ones; and when
you have laboriously accomplished your
daily task, go to sleep in peace.

— Victor Hugo

Life is something to do when you can't get
to sleep.

— Fran Lebowitz

We sleep, but the loom of life never stops,
and the pattern which was weaving when
the sun went down is weaving when it
comes up in the morning.

— Henry Ward Beecher

Leisure time is that five or six hours when
you sleep at night.

— George Allen, Sr.

The man who says his evening prayer is a
captain posting his sentinels. He can sleep.

— Charles Baudelaire

The main facts in human life are five: birth,
food, sleep, love and death.

— E.M. Forster

When I prayed for success, I forgot to ask
for sound sleep and good digestion.

— Mason Cooley

If I feel in need of sleep, I just open a book
or turn on the television. Both are better
than any sleeping pill.

— Ethel Merman

I no longer teach law. But when I did I
advised my students that they should never
accept a case if it meant that by doing so
you couldn't sleep at night.

— Christopher Darden

~

I.

The Prophets Want Profits

When I was first diagnosed with sleep apnea in November 1999 they told me I would need to use a CPAP system which consisted of a CPAP machine, tube and mask.

When I first saw these items, my reaction was, "There is no way I can sleep with that mask on. Wrestling with the tube and the noise of the machine will drive my wife nuts." I traveled a lot with my son and I figured the noise would keep him up.

The first step was getting fitted with a mask. There are many types of masks, and I do not recall the first ones they tried to fit me with. They gave me many to try on but none seemed to fit such that there would be no leak. After close to a half hour, I could see the technician getting frustrated because he was spending so much time with one patient and getting nowhere.

Often he would say, "Well that looks like it fits OK." To which I kept replying, "No, it does not fit. See ...." and I pointed out to him where it did not fit the contour of my face.

By that time I had tried on pretty much their entire inventory. Finally, he said he would try an entirely different mask system. He found that an Ultra Mirage II mask system – size large worked. It fitted me ok.

I do not mean to say, or imply, that this mask system will work for any of you. Each of our face contours is different. My point here is be tenacious. Be persistent. Do *not* leave until you have a mask that fits well. If I had not been so persistent, I would have been sent home with one of the other systems which fitted somewhat but not well.

You should not have any appreciable leakage. If the mask is not fitted correctly so that there are no leaks no matter what you do later, the system will not work for you. Many people have complained to me that their mask does not fit or fit well. I tell them to go back and don't leave until it fits satisfactorily. *Don't try and make due with a mask that does not fit well.*

I was given the mask, a box with the CPAP and a booklet and told it is easy, just read the book about use and care. The sleep clinic not only makes money on the sleep study, but also as the vendor of the equipment. It was apparent to me that they had little or no familiarity with the equipment because they never had to use it. If you can find a vendor who has an employee who has sleep apnea, they will better understand your problems and therefore be better able to help you.

Saying "Here is your mask, tube, your CPAP machine and a booklet. Good luck," is not satisfactory service and is not what you need. You need more information about how to make the equipment to work for you.

Read the booklet which came with your CPAP machine thoroughly. If there is a booklet with your mask system, you need to read that thoroughly also. It is my understanding from some of those who have attended my sleep apnea/CPAP classes that some mask systems come in a plastic bag with no instructions or booklet.

If yours does not have an instruction booklet, some questions you may want to ask your vendor are:

- How often should I wash the mask system?

- Do I need to take it apart each time I wash it?

- What cleaning agent should I use to wash it?

- How often should I wash the tube?

- What cleaning agent should I use to wash it?

- How do I dry the tube when it is washed?

- Do I need to wash the humidifier if I use only distilled water?

- If so, how often should I wash the humidifier?

- If so, what cleaning agent should I use to wash it?

- Should I use the humidifier year around or only when I am in places where the furnace is on?

~

II.

The BIG Secret

The BIG secret came to me after only a few days of use because when I slept and turned from side to side, the tube became tangled in the bedding and when tangled, it pulled on the mask breaking the seal. It occurred to me that if the tube were to hang down from above me, there was no way it could get tangled in the bedding.

The BIG Secret has two parts. This is the thing that really made CPAP work easily for me.

(1) *THE TUBE MUST HANG DOWN FROM ABOVE YOUR HEAD* [2]
(2) *USE AN ELASTIC SYSTEM TO HOLD THE TUBE.*

---

[2] To better enable the reader to understand how this works pictures are set forth in Chapter XV (*see* Pictures #1–10).

Pictures #1 and 2 (p.71) show the system I developed at home. By having the tube hang down from above where your head is when you sleep, when you turn over regardless of which side, the tube never gets caught, never bothers you and you don't really know it is there. In addition, and very importantly the tube *does not pull on the mask* as it would if it was lying on or in the bedding. Picture #2 (p.71) shows that regardless of which side I am on, the tube will not get caught. Because the system hanging down is elastic, the tube follows me where I turn.

Most users are fine when you sleep on the side facing the table/machine. However, when the tubing does not hang down from above, there is a problem when you sleep on your back or face away from the CPAP generator. Then, the tubing must lie on top of you and it often gets caught in the bedding or your arms. This pulls on the tubing and can twist the mask on your face and break the seal. By hanging the tubing down from above you, these problems are solved.

If you use a six-foot tube, that will be plenty of length. What I did was put a hook in the ceiling like that which is used for hanging plants. See Pictures #1 and 2 (p.71).

I then hung a two-foot bungee cord from the hook. The last foot or two is a string of rubber bands. Rubber bands work well because they move and are flexible. The bungee cord is not needed and you can in fact just use a string of rubber bands from the ceiling hook to the level you want. From experience I find that a double row of rubber bands works best (*see* Picture #1, p.71).

Others have come to the same conclusion that the best way to use CPAP is to have the tube come down from above you rather than wrap around you. There are some products on the Internet[3] that accomplish the same thing but at a greater expense and more difficulty when you travel. There is really nothing cheaper and easier to

---

[3] I am not providing Internet links because from experience I have found that often by the time the reader checks the links they are dead links. Insetad I will provide a generic description which permits the reader to find products which fit the function. Newer products will also be found this way.

transport than rubber bands which are free if you use the ones that come around your mail each day. If you need to purchase them, the cost is nominal. Further, it is much easier to take rubber bands with you when you travel.

There is really nothing cheaper and easier to transport than the rubber bands which are free if you use the ones that come around your mail each day. If you need to purchase them, the cost is nominal. Further, it is much easier to take rubber bands with you when you travel and nothing works better.

For those of you who do not want, or can't, put a hook in the ceiling above where you head goes on the pillow, there are other ways to get the tube to hang down from above you. You can put a hook or nail in the wall above your head. If you can't do that because there is a picture or something else on the wall above your head, then you can hang the rubber bands from that. This is the method I use when I travel.

When you travel, you do not need to put a hook in the ceiling above you. There are much easier ways to get the tube to hang down from above you depending on a number of factors which will be discussed in the chapter on "Traveling Made Easier."

~

III.

Little Secrets

To effectively use CPAP your nasal system must be clear to breathe and not be plugged because of a cold or allergy nor blocked by nasal polyps.

My nasal septum was not straight and, in addition, I had a number of nasal polyps that inhibited the air flow of my breathing. Both problems were taken care of during nasal surgery. Now I breathe better both during the day and at night. In addition, now CPAP works much better for me.

For nasal stuffiness I suggest using AFRIN® nasal spray, it works great. AFRIN® nasal spray is a nonprescription item. It is what is used by many radiologists when they need to X-ray your nasal and sinus areas. It is important to follow the directions of not to use for more than three days.

For those of you with allergies especially to dust mites, there are a number of things you can do depending on the severity of your allergy. One thing that works quite well is to use an allergy mattress and box spring cover. This creates a physical barrier to prevent the allergen from reaching you. Second, you can get allergy shots. I have an allergy to mold which creates real problems for me in the fall. To prevent this mold allergy from being a problem in my life, I chose to receive allergy shots. As long as I had to make the trip to the allergist's office and get stuck, the injected cocktail also had medication to treat the dust mite allergy.

I found the allergy shots worked wonders for me, and I recommend you seriously consider taking to your physician about getting them if your allergy is causing you a problem. Alternatively, or in addition, you may want to use an antihistamine at bedtime. Many antihistamines do not require a prescription and are OTC[4]. The major side effect of most OTC antihistamines is drowsiness. But if you are going to bed it is not an issue. For those of you who are still drowsy in the morning

---

[4] OTC is Over The Counter: it does not require a prescription.

from the antihistamine, there are newer prescription antihistamines which do not cause drowsiness.

For those who are congested because of colds, an OTC decongestant like SUDAFED® tablets works well. The 12- or 24-hour versions work all night.

There is another very neat item that makes CPAP life much easier. For some reason I have never found another CPAP user that is aware of it. However, after I show them how easy it makes attaching the mask and tube or tube and CPAP, virtually everyone says they are going to get it. I found that when I got up at night to use the restroom, I had to twist and fight with the tube to separate it from the mask piece.

Worse yet, upon return from the restroom, I had to fight with the tube to get it to firmly attach to the appropriate piece on the mask. After a night or two of this fighting, I recalled that in organic chemistry lab we had ground glass joints which permitted one piece of glassware to attach to another with no effort and no pushing; the two pieces just slid together. There is a similar product for connecting the tube to the mask and tube to the CPAP but made out of hard plastic, see Picture #10 (p.76) These connectors can be purchased from most stores selling CPAP supplies or on-line and usually come in pairs.

They make detaching your tube so easy I have often done it with one hand.

~

IV.

Changing Tires

You would not leave home in your car without a spare tire for the car, so why would you leave home with out a spare fuse for your CPAP?

My old machine had a fuse, my new one does not. You should check your machine to see if it has a replaceable fuse. If so, find out the kind and requirements and get a spare to keep in your travel bag. The cost is nominal.

In March 2007 I arrived in London for vacation with plans to go to France and Belgium. Upon landing and arriving at the hotel and getting my room I began to hook up my BiPAP. To make sure it would operate on the European 220 (it was supposed to), I tried it. It would not turn on. After some checking, I determined it was the fuse. Being in the UK where they only have metric items, I don't know if I could have found a replacement fuse for my machine. But because I always had a spare or two in my bag it was not an issue.

Think of it like taking a spare tire; don't leave home without a spare fuse. In addition, having one even at home can be very helpful. If you do not go to bed until late and you find you need a new fuse, there may be no stores open at that time. It is best to always keep a spare tire in the bag.

Besides having a spare fuse, it is prudent to have spare parts for your mask. It may be possible for you to purchase them or even a back up mask. But the easiest, best and cheapest way to do this is to *save your old masks*. Depending on your insurance company you may be able to get a new mask every six months or every year or ??? But when ever you do, do *not* discard the old one. Wash it, dry it, put it in a plastic bag and put it in a box on the shelf. From my experience over the past decade of use, I can guarantee[5] you will now and then find

---

[5] While finalizing this book the little plastic tab on the elastic head straps that holds the mask to the head gear broke off. I

that those spare parts come in very handy when you break some piece or lose it. The mask parts are plastic and can and do break. It is also possible that as you wash them, one of the small ones may go down the drain. It will be easier to replace it than to take the drain apart. With my kids' contacts, I had to take the drain apart and I can tell you from experience, it is much easier to keep spare parts.

Similarly, when you get a new tube, save the old one. Here there is not as much of a problem with tubes as with masks. With tubes, electrical tape can usually easily repair a crack that occurs and will do the job well and take up less space than a backup tube.

For snowbirds who head from the snowy north to the warm sunny south in the winter, I strongly recommend taking the spare parts with you. While it is possible to get a mask or parts where you go in the south, how do you know they stock parts for the particular mask that you have? Once I left a part at home and needed one

---

went to my box of spare parts and replaced it with the corresponding piece from my last mask.

when in Tennessee. There was only one
dealer that I could find that carried the type
of mask I use and had the part I needed.
For short vacations I do not take spare
parts with me. If something breaks, I will
use glue. If I will be gone a few weeks or
more, I will consider taking spare parts.
They are very light and take up very little
room. The tube takes up considerably more
room, but most any problem with a tube
can be fixed with electrical or duct tape and
that should not be too difficult to find.

~

V.

Bathing Regularly

I am sure you are all well aware that you need to wash your mask daily and the tube as the manufacturer recommends. Just as the manufacturer of a car recommends oil changes probably more regularly than needed, so too with CPAP equipment. I am not going to tell any of you to do other than what your manufacturer recommends. You should follow the manufacturer's recommendations. I will only tell you what I do.

With regard to the mask, each day I completely disassemble, soak in hot soap (IVORY® soap) solution for about 10–15 min. I then rinse each part and set them out to dry on a paper towel in the bowl that I used to wash them in. At night just before I am going to bed, when they are dry I reassemble. A substantial number of people in the course I teach do not dissemble the mask but wash it as one piece. If that is what your manufacturer recommends, fine. My concern in doing that with my mask system is that because of all the pieces and small crevices I am not sure I could get the soapy solution into all the places it needs to be. Because there are a number of different mask systems, your's may be such that it can readily be washed with out disassembling.

Further, I doubt that if I washed mine in one piece it would be dry by night time. There are many very small spaces or crevices that it would be difficult for air to get into to dry it.

With regard to the tube, some manufacturers recommend washing daily. For almost 11 years, I have washed mine once a week using the same type of soap solution I use for washing the mask. I rinse and dry in the same manner.

For those of you who use a humidifier and need to have a jacket around your tube to keep the water vapor from condensing, there are two ways to wash the tube. You can either remove the jacket or wash it with the jacket on. Often this depends on how easy it is to remove the jacket as explained below.

Regarding washing and drying the tube, I will pass along some information provided to me by an ear, nose and throat (ENT) physician. He told me that he thought I should be running alcohol through my tube regularly to make sure it did not house any bacteria. I am not exactly sure what he meant by "regularly" (weekly or monthly?) but since I had used CPAP for about six years at that point split between two different tubes with absolutely no problem, I have not done that at the frequency he recommended. Now, I run alcohol through it about once every six months. You can use either ethyl alcohol or isopropyl alcohol for this purpose. When you do, you should hook it up and blow air through the tubing for a minute or two to get the alcohol vapor out of the tubing before attaching it to your mask.

Insurance companies differ in how often they will cover a new mask and/or tubing. I have used masks for more than two years and tubes for almost five years before replacing. I don't recommend that, but I mention it only to show that with regular cleaning I have used both the mask system and tube for longer periods than recommended without a problem. I am convinced that if I had to use my mask system for a third or even fourth year, it probably would have been ok. So for those of you without insurance take real good care of your mask parts by washing daily and you should be able to use them for a considerable period.

Please remember I am not recommending in any way that you do other than what the manufacturer of your mask system and tube tells you to do.

~

VI.

Humidifiers

Humidity is the measure of water in the air. Generally, warmer air can hold more moisture and cold air is capable of holding much less. Humidity is expressed as a percent of the maximum moisture air can contain.

Humidifiers are not only useful but really necessary in the northern climates where in late fall, winter and early spring furnaces are used for heat. The humidity of a house where the outside temperature is 20° F (-7° C) can not get very high because if it does, the humidity will condense on the cold windows reducing the moisture content of the air and keeping the inside humidity low. The colder the outside temperature, the lower will be the humidity inside. There is no correlation chart for outside temperature and inside humidity because the amount of humidity the inside air will handle at any given outside temperature will vary depending on (1) the amount of surface area of your windows and (2) how well insulated your windows are. Low humidity dries out your nose and lungs. Use of CPAP with low humidity can dry out your mucous membranes increasing the risk of bleeding and infection.

With the air blowing through a sleep-apneic individual's airways all night, the airways will get dried out and more susceptible to infection if humidity is not added.

To deal with the low room humidity, CPAP machines can be connected to a humidifier. Actually many newer models now come with either a built in humidifier or one that attaches easily to the main CPAP unit. In either event, if you are in the snow belt or even close, it is best to use a humidifier. I spent last winter in Tampa and did not need my humidifier there because the night time outside temperature was generally in the 40s to 50s with relatively high humidity.

The humidifier manufacturers will tell you how often to wash those units. You should follow those directions. I use only *distilled* water in my humidifier and have never ever washed it. In the morning, I pour out the remaining water and put the pieces in a drawer (so little or no dust will get at it) and let them dry. In the evening, I reassemble, add *distilled* water and use it. Distilled water by definition has nothing in it so when it evaporates there is absolutely nothing left. All other water will have some residue when the water evaporates. Regardless of how often you wash your humidifier, I suggest using distilled water in it.

I remember the first time I used my humidifier. I turned it on and I could feel that the air had some humidity but was cold. As the heater increased the temperature of the water, more moisture came over. I fell asleep. ZZZZZZZZZZZZZZZ Sometime later I woke up thinking I was drowning with water running down my nostrils and all over the mask. I quickly got up and realized the problem was that the water was heating nicely in the humidifier, vaporizing up the tube, but when it reached that part of the tube where the temperature was sufficiently low, it would condense on the sides of the tube.

We keep our bedroom temperature at about 65° at night. The humidifier adds moisture and warms the air. If the tubing does not prevent the warm moist air from cooling, the drop in temperature results in condensation (the forming of water droplets because the amount of moisture exceeds what the now cooler air can hold). When there was enough condensate, the water droplets would run down and into my schnoz! The humidifier was working efficiently at distilling over the water vapor which then condensed as distillate in my nose. Dummy!

The easy solution is to keep the tube warm enough so the moist air will not condense. The way to do that is to put an insulating coat or sheath around the tube.

Many commercial sheaths, jackets, socks or wraps do exist. Eleven years ago when I first started to use BiPAP, I was unaware of the commercial tube jackets so I went to the local fabric store and purchased sufficient insulating material to cover six feet of tube and then contracted with someone there to run one seam up for me. Dummy! Now, how do I get the tube to crawl inside all the way to the other end? You can't just push it through; it is limp!

Some commercial tube coverings have a zipper; that works well. Mine didn't. What I did was take a sturdy coat hanger, open it up, put a loop on the end and attached a long string. I then worked the coat hanger through the sheath until I could grab the coat hanger at the other end and pull the rope through. Once the rope is through I made a noose, put it around the tubing and pulled the tubing through. When I wanted to remove the tubing for its weekly bath, I put the noose around one end of the tubing and when I pulled the tubing out of the sheath, the rope is left in the sheath ready to pull the tubing back when it was dry. Since then I have learned to wash the tubing without having to remove it from the sheath. My homemade sheath is shown in Pictures #1, 2 and 4 through 8 (pp.71,72–75). There are numerous commercial sheaths on the market which are much slimmer than mine, see Picture #3 (p.72).

If you use a humidifier you will need to cover the tubing with some sort of sheath.

Fisher Paykel makes thermosmart heated hoses for some of their units so a sheath is not needed.

ResMed S9 series has a H5i humidifier with ClimateLine tubing that is also heated. Respironics System One has redesigned humidity system to reduce rainout.

Don't make a sheath for your tube (even one even with a zipper in it). It will probably cost about the same to purchase one and you will have much less work. The only reason I did not initially purchase one is that I was unaware they were commercially available.

Some of those who have used a sheath or tube covers have reported two adverse consequences. The first is that it makes the tube stiffer and the second is it adds weight. Both are expected consequences of adding a sheath for insulation but neither is sufficient reason to prevent use of the sheath. However, if you use my system of hanging the tube down from a hook in the ceiling above you by an elastic bungee cord/rubber band system, the problem with increased weight is completely dealt with as the elastic system holds the tube regardless of the weight. The increased stiffness is there but because the elastic system is very flexible and moveable, virtually all of the stiffness is eliminated.

While using the humidifier is a little more work, it is worth it in keeping your nasal area moist when the humidity is low inside. I suggest at least trying the humidifier for a week and then you can compare and see what works best for you. You will also learn which setting on the humidifier works best for you. I suggest starting with a low setting and increasing it rather than starting with a high setting and working your way down.

~

VII.

Part A – Traveling Made Easier (In General)

Whether you travel a little or a lot – on vacation or for buisiness or to visit relatives, you need to take your CPAP with you *every time you go*. It is the first thing I pack.

First a list of things to take and then I will explain the reason for each:

Extra fuses

Foreign adapters

Plug for electric outlets that are not grounded

Plug increasing outlets from 1 to 3

Extension cord

Strings of rubber bands

Bag of extra rubber bands

Small container with:
Nails
Hooks

> Suction stick on hooks
> Picture hangers

Flexible wash container (travel)

Meds – antihistamine, decongestant, nasal spray

The first thing to do when traveling outside of the United States is to check the booklet that came with your CPAP to determine if your machine can run on 220 v (often outside of the United States) as well as 110 v (United States). If not, you will need a converter. Most newer units run on both.

The reason for the extra fuses has already been explained. Having a spare one in London saved my two-week vacation.

Different countries have different outlets. The standard three pronged plug that we have here in the U.S. does not fit the outlets in many countries. If you travel outside of the U.S., purchase a standard bag of adapters for foreign travel. This bag will have an adapter for virtually any country you will travel to. You need not take this bag with you if you are only traveling in the U.S. or on most cruise liners.

The plug for electric outlets that are not grounded is for older buildings which only have the old two pronged receptacles. These outlets will not handle the three prongs of most CPAP units. I have been told by some that their CPAP machines only have two pronged plugs. If yours has only two prongs, then this is not an issue for you.

The plug increasing outlets from one to three is very useful if you need to charge a cell phone, a camera battery, your laptop *and* run your CPAP. I have used this fairly often, especially in Europe where there are not as many outlets as in the U.S.

The extension cord probably needs no explanation. A small one of eight or ten feet is sufficient.

The strings of rubber bands are to get the tube to hang down from above you. I carry two strings with me. The longest is about seven or eight feet and the short one is about three feet. Using just these two strings of rubber bands, there are only two occasions where I could not get things to work without some additional modification. One was in St. Louis where the headboard was an immense old European one going all the way to the ceiling. Usually the large strand is strung horizontally, usually over the edges of a picture or pictures above the headboard. The short one is then strung over the horizontal one, usually double stranded, and it hangs down. It is very easy to adjust the height by using the appropriate rings of the rubber band ladder. If there is a headboard one can use the ends to attach the horizontal string of bands to.

Pictures #4 through #8 (pp.72–75) show how this works. These were taken at three local motels to demonstrate how I do this.

Pictures #4 and #5 (pp.72–73) illustrate the general concept of using two rubber band strings. In addition, these pictures demonstrate the use of a headboard when there are no pictures.

Picture #6 (p.74) illustrates the general concept of using two rubber band strings when a picture is present. There is a headboard, but it is probably too low to be used effectively.

Pictures #7 and #8 (p.75) also illustrate how a little creativity is helpful. There is no picture above the bed, but there are two wall hangings that can be used to span the horizontal rubber band string.

Picture #8 (p.75) illustrates an alternative way of hanging the vertical strand. To do this the wall hangings are not used. The vertical strand is hung from the light fixture.

Picture #9 (p.76) illustrates how the rubber band system can be used where there is no convenient wall or ceiling to hang the rubber band system from. Here I used a (extendable) pole for washing windows.

I carry extra rubber bands with me in case one or more break or I need to add length to one of the two strands. Occasionally a third strand has been useful.

The small container holds assorted items of nails, hooks, suction stick on hooks and picture hangers so you are prepared if there is nothing on the wall above the bed for you to hook the rubber bands to. This happens about ten percent of the time. When it does, you can use one of the items in the container to attach to the wall so you have something to hook the vertical rubber band string on. When you do this, the horizontal string is not needed.

During the past decade or so I have traveled to England, France, Australia, New

Zealand, Alaska, Spain and Canada and gone on two cruises. In addition, I have been to about 40 states at least once and many several times. I mention this only because in all these travels only once have I not been able to get my system hooked up with the items I set forth above. The other time I was not able to get the two rubber band system to operate easily was downtown Chicago where there was nothing on the wall for me to attach the (horizontal) rubber band string to. In addition, the wall was true plaster and I could not get any of my hooks, nails of picture frame holders into the wall. So I went to the Walgreens pharmacy on the corner of Chicago Ave and N. Michigan Ave and purchased a roll of duct tape which I used to adhere one of my hooks to the wall. Victory!

On one other occasion I could not get the picture hanger in the wall and borrowed a hammer from the motel "maintenance engineer."

Three times during the past decade I required surgery which necessitated an overnight stay in the hospital. On each occasion *Barbara* made the trip with me. If you are having surgery it is critical that you let your surgeon and anesthesiologist know that you have sleep apnea and use CPAP. The reason is you may need it in recovery after receiving sedation or anesthesia. Your CPAP should go with you were ever you travel with very few exceptions.

The one place I did not take it was when I hiked to the bottom of the Grand Canyon. It was just too heavy to carry down and up. There are burros that take down supplies for the lodge at the bottom and they will take it for you but they want it a day ahead of time. In hindsight, I made the wrong decision. It would have been best not to have it the one night before I went down but have it at the bottom before the hike out since it is much more strenuous coming up. For those of you who may take that beautiful hike, I recommend having the burro take it down so you have it when you are down there. In addition, most hikers stay two nights at the bottom (I recommend this also), and you will only miss one night not having it at the top.

What do you wash your mask in when you travel? If you are staying at a motel/hotel, you can usually use the ice bucket of the motel/hotel. If you are staying with relative you can use any small container they have in the kitchen. Because I travel a lot I used to take a TUPPERWARE® bowl with me in my suitcase stuffed with underwear or something. The airlines broke three or four of these. A friend who likes to cook told me to try a CHEFMATE® baking pan. It's great. It's unbreakable. I use a 9 x 5 one. The neat thing is that the CHEFMATE® baking pans are made of some type of rubber that is flexible. There is no way anyone can break it. I have had this one for about five years with absolutely no problems.

Washing your mask when traveling can be a little different. This occurs when you have to travel very early in the morning and there is no time to let the mask components air dry. In those circumstances, I hand dry the pieces with a paper towel or something similar. Then when I pack the pieces except the flexible plastic piece that fits against the face, I put them in a mesh bag so any remaining moisture in these pieces can evaporate while I am traveling. The flexible plastic piece that fits against the face I put in a hard plastic container to protect it and then cover with a piece of mesh so it too can air dry any remaining moisture.

This procedure evolved over the period of a decade while traveling to Europe, New Zealand/Australia, about 40 states and two cruises. Picture #11 (p.77) shows the eight plastic pieces on the left with the mesh bag at the top. On the right is the flexible plastic piece that goes against the face. Above it is the hard plastic piece which houses this when it is packed. Picture #12 (p.77) shows the mesh bag containing the eight pieces and the hard plastic container with the flexible mask piece ready to be packed.

Make sure you take any medications with you that you use at home.

When flying, *NEVER EVER CHECK YOUR CPAP.* The airports screeners are used to seeing them and they are too important to you to not take as a carry on. It can get lost permanently or be damaged if it is checked. Even if it is not lost permanently or damaged, if it gets sent to the wrong city you may be without it for a day or two before it gets back to you.

Part B - Traveling Made Easier
(Cars, Campers, Boats)

When staying in a motel, hotel or relatives home we assume the power supply is the same as at home. That is a valid assumption.

However, that is not always the situation with campers and motor homes and never the situation with cars. With campers and motor homes they can supply alternating current (AC) if they are at a camp site which has an electrical power hookup or if a generator is used. Boats can supply AC if they have a generator. However, if the camper, motor home or boat is not supplied with external power, and you use the vehicles battery – you will be getting direct current (DC).

What kind of current does your CPAP or BiPAP machine use? It depends on your machine. Mine can use either AC or DC. All will operate on AC and some only on AC. A friend's CPAP operates on DC (it has an inverter in the line to convert AC to DC). The best way to know what type of current you machine uses is to check your manual.

If your machine is of the type that only uses AC and you want to use the battery of a car, camper, motor home or boat you will need to get an inverter. You will also need to know the number of amps that your machine draws to determine how many watts are required. Inverters can be purchased on-line or in a variety of retail stores.

The question arises if you want to spend the night in your car at a rest stop, will the battery last all night and if so, will it have sufficient power to start the car in the morning. I will give an attorney's answer, "It depends!" It depends on the strength of your battery, the length of time you have your machine on, the amount of current your machine will draw, etc. I have never used a battery to power my machine which uses five amps of 12 volt DC. However, a friend whose machine draws three amps used a 12 volt battery for two nights without a problem.

My recommendation is, if it is possible, do a dry run. Hook your CPAP up to the vehicle, whatever it may be, and let it run 7–8 hours. Then check and see if the battery has enough power to start the vehicle. If it does, during the next day's travel, the generator will recharge the car's battery so you will have sufficient power for your CPAP for the following night.

~

VIII.

Nap Time

Probably the most critical or dangerous problem resulting from sleep apnea is the lack of oxygen to the tissues. However, those with sleep apnea do not sense that. The thing that most individuals with sleep apnea complain about is being tired or exhausted. That was my big complaint before I was diagnosed with sleep apnea.

The excessive tiredness results not from not getting enough sleep (total hours) but from not getting good quality (REM sleep). One way those with sleep apnea try and deal with the problem of excessive tiredness is to catch a nap when they can.

Before I was diagnosed with sleep apnea my son was doing competitive skiing. Many of the larger meets were in northern Michigan and required a 3–6 hour drive. Often I was so tired, I was afraid I would fall asleep while driving and would have to pull over and take a nap. When my wife and I went together, she would drive and I would sleep.

I recall my dad, who unquestionably had sleep apnea, taking naps on the weekend. As a teenager I could not figure why an adult would want to sleep during the day. Now I know.

The material with my BiPAP informed me that if I napped, that I should use the BiPAP when I napped. I think that is good advice for the usual weekend nap of a couple of hours. I don't use it because my naps are all less than 30 minutes as explained below.

There are a number of different ways to "nap" and I have found some are better than others for me. Most individuals nap only on weekends and their nap time is usually at least one hour and can last several hours. Often when I woke up from multi-hour naps, I was groggy and did not feel any more refreshed than when I laid down.

There is another way to nap which I learned from my wife who was born and raised in Taiwan. She did not come to the U.S. until she entered graduate school.

Both her parents were principals in their respective school systems. In Taiwan after lunch everyone (all students and teachers included) takes a 30 min nap; it is considered part of the school day.

The Asian way of "napping" is a very short nap time, usually about 20–30 min. When I first tried this I went past the half-hour marker still zzzzzzzzzzzzzzzzzzzzz. So I started setting the alarm on my watch for 20—25 min. After a period of about a year, I noticed many times I would get up just before the alarm went off. I then moved the alarm to 30 min and found that almost always was I woke up before the alarm went off. Amazingly, I found these very short naps left me very refreshed.

There is another important aspect in taking the short nap. That is, where it is taken. I found that if I lay down on a soft area like my bed or couch, it was pretty easy to go past 30 min. However, if I napped in a place that was not like night sleeping I very rarely went past the 30 min mark; usually between 22–30 min. Once you get the hang of putting your head down and taking a nap with people around it is easy. For example, various places I have taken naps that are unlike my bed are: putting my head down on the desk; in airplanes; after lunch going out to my car[6]; Centennial Park in Atlanta during the 1996 Olympics; between the two tennis stadiums in Indianapolis during a break in the Davis Cup tournament matches; after receiving an allergy shot and being told to wait 30 min in the waiting room (perfect time and place for a nap); in the car when my wife or son is driving; in vacant offices at work, in some large park in Sydney, Australia; in New Zealand while riding on tour buses when there is nothing to see and it is just transportation; on a train in Alaska when going from Denali to Fairbanks and not much to see; etc.

The interesting question is how short of a nap will help. I don't know the absolute answer but it is probably between five and ten minutes for me. I will offer observations

---

[6] I am aware that there is good advice not to nap in a car. The reason is you should not get use to falling asleep in a place where you may need to stay awake. When I nap I put the seat back, tilt the backrest back and to me it is much different than driving. I have done this for >10 yrs.

to substantiate this which I found by accident.

I used to take my son for swimming lessons at the YMCA when he was about two years old. Because we lived about 30 minutes from town, I would pick him up from daycare and we would go to the Burger King for a quick dinner because it was less than a mile from the Y. When we were done with dinner, I would put him in his car seat and drive over the Y. Often he would fall asleep on the ride over. I would let him sleep as long as I could before getting him up and into the Y. He usually had a 5–15 minute nap. The difference in his personality was like night and day even with at the short end of the interval. I was very surprised that such a short nap would help. So I decided to try it.

On many occasions when I am tired and have only a short time before a meeting, golf game or something I must due and the possibility is there for a nap, I do the following: I take the time I have available before the meeting (maybe 15 minutes) subtract 5 minutes and set my cell phone for 10 minutes from the present time. It works great! I am relaxed about not missing the event because of the alarm on my cell phone. The 5 or 10 minutes of "nap" that I get is awesome. I can't believe how much better I feel – almost as if I had the entire 25 minute "quickie."

I am a patent attorney by trade. In the afternoon many times if I am reading, my eyes close and then I have trouble remembering what I read. So I go back and reread what I read before and guess what – my eyes usually close again! Not very efficient or productive. So I go and take a short nap. My increased efficiency after that more than makes up for the time I took to nap. Often because of meetings, these naps are limited to 5–15 min but are well worth it.

Because it works so well for me, I tend to "nap" probably six days a week on the average. Sometimes it will be earlier like 1:30 or later like 5:00. It will be at different places such as the allergist office or my car. One word of caution; if you take your nap late in the day some people have trouble going to bed at their usual bed time. Since we tend to go to bed late (12:00am to 1:00am] taking a late nap is not a problem for me.

When you are tired and have the opportunity of taking a nap, do it. Just set some sort of alarm for 25 minutes. If you only have 20 minutes, take a 15-minute nap. I am sure you will feel much better.

For those of you who do not have sleep apnea and are reading this book for some reason, I highly recommend that you too try the "quickie."

~

IX.

Who Turned The Lights Off?

We have all had the experience of going to bed at night and in the morning realizing the alarm did not go off because during the night the power had gone off. Hopefully, you were not late for a plane or missed some important meeting.

What happens in those situations to CPAP users? Simple, no power—no CPAP. Your machine goes off and you are awakened. You take off your mask and have to sleep the rest of the night without the benefits of CPAP. Sometimes you are aware the power is back on. At that point you can put your mask back on and restart your CPAP machine. The time you were without CPAP can be a few minutes to many hours.

Many of you have had the experience of working on your computer when a power outage occurred. Probably many or most of you have a UPS (Uninterruptible Power

Supply) which provides sufficient power to your computer for a few minutes so you can save your documents and shut your system down in an orderly way. Will this type of system work at night for your CPAP? I will give a lawyers answer, yes and no! Yes, it can power your CPAP as it powers your computer. No, because while it powers your computer, it does so only for a short period of time, usually five to fifteen minutes, so you can save the documents you were working on. It does not have sufficient power to run your computer for a prolonged period of time or your CPAP for the rest of the night.

You can try and protect against a power outage by having a long talk with the man with the long white beard upstairs. Otherwise I suggest looking for a UPS with a long back up time. There are commercially available ones that last for "up to five hours."

An alternative to finding a commercially ready made one is to have an electrician build you one using a car battery so you will have sufficient power to get through the night in the event the power goes out early in the evening. My eldest son has built one for me. It works well. In the 11 years I have used BiPAP we have lost power about a handful of times and it has worked each time. In fact, when we lose power I don't even know it until the next morning. I just keep sleeping as if there was no power outage because for my BiPAP there was no power outage.

~

X.

Learning to Count

Whether you count one, two, three, four
(English); אחד, שתיים, שלוש, ארבע (Hebrew); or
uno, dos, tres, cuatro (Spanish); or using
your fingers and toes, it is important with
regard to CPAP for two different reasons as
explained below.

The two reasons are (1) when you
disassemble and wash your mask, not to
lose a piece and (2) when you pack your
CPAP for travel not to leave a piece behind.

When you wash your mask, I recommend
disassembling it, soaking it in soapy water
for a few minutes (I do this while I shave)
and then rinse each piece and set to dry.
One night when I first started using BiPAP
and went to reassemble the mask, I noticed
that one of the small parts was missing. In
hindsight I realized that I had missed
taking it out of the washbowl to rinse and
then dumped it down the drain with the

wash water. Now when I take the pieces out of the washbowl to rinse off, I count each one. I don't dump the wash water until all parts are accounted for. My old mask assembly had ten; this one only has nine. From experience, I can tell you it is much easier to count the pieces than to take the drain trap assembly apart.

When you take your CPAP for a vacation and you pack your travel bag you need to include the CPAP machine, the power cord (mine has two pieces), the tube, all the parts of your mask parts, a small bottle of soap, and anything else you deem necessary, see the Chapter on travel.

In the morning when I wash my mask, I do not wash the elastic material and plastic piece that attaches to the mask assembly and holds it to your head. I just hang that on a hook and at night after the mask itself is assembled, I attach it to the elastic head band. Years ago when I had to leave town on business, I washed the mask in the usually manner, dried each piece since there was no time to air dry and packed my bag to go see the wonderful world of Mississippi. That night after I assembled my mask I went to attach it to the elastic head band but only to realize that it was hanging on the hook about 800 miles away in Kalamazoo. That night I used rubber bands to make an elastic head band assembly. It worked, but not well. My wife overnighted the wayward piece to me. Now I count all the pieces when I pack to make sure I have everything. Again, from experience, I can tell you it is much easier to count the pieces when you pack than to try and make due at the other end. Fortunately, the elastic head band assembly is something that you can "make do" with rubber bands or some other means of holding the mask to your head. However, some of the other items like power cord or tube – you will be up the creek without the canoe.

~

XI.

What's in A Name?

Different individuals have very different sensitivities about others knowing about their medical conditions including sleep apnea.

When traveling through airports or on trains, it is hard to disguise your CPAP bag. However, non-CPAP users will not recognize the "CPAP bag" because they are not familiar with it. Usually only other "users" will recognize it.

One way not to call attention to your CPAP in public is by giving it a name or identifying word. Any name or word you and your family agree on is fine.

Another reason is just convenience. It is much easier to refer to a one word identifier than "your breathing machine" or "your BiPAP" or "the breathing machine" or etc. I chose Barbara as a fitting name for my BiPAP.

If I had a CPAP I probably would have called it Carol for fun and convenience.

One website which sells tube socks to cover the tubes suggests giving the tube sock a name; the name they suggest is Paul!

~

XII.

Family

One concern that individuals with sleep apnea have is, "How is my using CPAP going to affect my family?" Certainly a valid and important question. Fortunately and surprisingly, the answer is positively.

Most all who have sleep apnea snore and the snoring is disruptive of sleep of those in the same room as they. I could hear my dad down the hall. I don't know if he woke me or I awoke for some other reason and heard him. I am surprised that we did not get calls from neighbors blocks away that my dad's snoring was disturbing their households.

If one uses CPAP successfully, the snoring will be replaced by the hum of the CPAP. That hum drowns out other annoying sounds. Both my wife and son are used to the sound. According to my son, "Barbara makes no more noise than if one had a fan in the room." My wife's comment is, "The steady humming noise is like white noise and easy to get used to."

One reviewer of this book is the wife of a CPAP user. Her comments are an excellent summary of how sleep apnea and CPAP can affect family:

> As the wife of a sleep apnea person, my sleep is severely compromised when my husband does not use his device or when he uses it without addressing some of the issues covered in this book.
>
> His mask emits a high pitch squeal when it doesn't fit properly or has pulled to one side because his hose gets caught in the bed linens. He does not use his sleep apnea device on trips which is an annoyance to other folks around him. When we stay at Hostels the management has to put us in a private room to avoid disturbing other guests—which isn't a bad

compromise—except that I
still cannot sleep even with
ear plugs.

I have asked others whether they
recommend ear plugs for those who sleep
in the same room as a CPAP user. The
answer uniformly is, "No, it's not needed."

Even if one is inclined not to use CPAP all
the time or when traveling, etc., you
should be aware that if you don't, it
adversely affects your significant other.
Isn't it better to wake up to a well rested,
smiling, happy significant other rather
than one who did not get a good night's
sleep and is tired and grouchy?

~

XIII.

Keeping Records

It is very important for you to keep good records of your sleep apnea diagnosis and treatment as well as when and where you get your supplies. The reason is that you will need to refer back to your sleep study and possibly produce a copy for insurance in order to get your supplies. If you have two or more sleep studies, especially if they are at different places and years apart, keeping copies of all records and a record of where, when and who will save you a lot of time in the long run.

If at times different doctors prescribe for you, you will need to have a record of who they are and how you can contact them.

Further, if your insurance permits a new mask at given intervals, such as one year, you will want to know when that year is up.

You can use any word processing system to keep just a simple record of the date, amount of funds involved and who/where/why. That way not only is everything in chronological order but you can electronically search for a particular doctor, vendor or any other information that you want to retrieve.

~

XIV.

Hear Ye! Hear Ye!

Hear ye! Hear ye!

When you will be sleeping in a room with individuals who are not familiar with sleep apnea/CPAP and/or who have never slept in a room with anyone with sleep apnea, you should explain to them in a few sentences what sleep apnea is and what "the machine" is for.

This serves two unrelated purposes. First, and foremost, is so those who are not familiar with CPAP will not be frightened or confused when everyone goes to bed. This way they will understand that "the machine" will make some background noise. This is a courtesy to those who will sleep in the room with you. They may ask that you let them get to sleep before you go to bed so the noise from the CPAP will not keep them from going to sleep. When my wife and I take a "quick" nap in the car, she often asks me to let her fall asleep before I put my head back because if I fall asleep first, often my snoring has kept her from falling asleep. The exception to this is if you are in a two-bed hospital room. Given all that is going on, I don't see a need for you to explain anything to the other person in the room.

The second purpose is for your benefit. If the people sleeping in the room with you understand the set-up, they can be of help to you. If during the night, they get up for any reason and realize that your mask has moved so that there is no seal and you are not getting the benefits of CPAP, they can wake and tell you. This permits you to reposition the mask. You sleep better and make less noise; a win-win situation. This will not happen unless they understand CPAP and feel they know you well enough to wake you.

~

XV.

Pictures

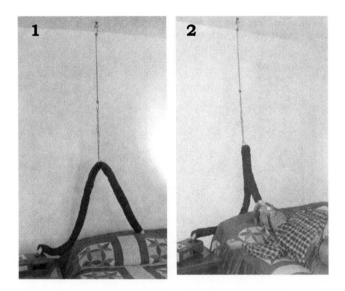

#1 – Home; this demonstrates the system.
See the hook in the ceiling, the 2' bungee cord
and a small double strand of rubber bands.
#2 – The author is on his right side.

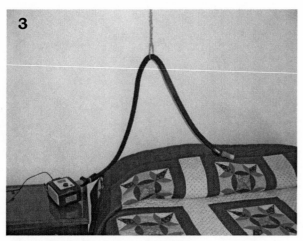

#3 − Thinner tube. Shown is a much thinner tube insulator than in picture #1. This one has a zipper.

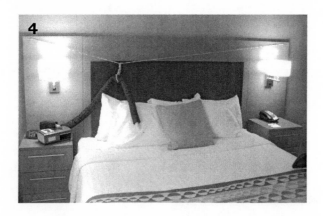

 # 4− Motel A. Here is the general concept of using two rubber band strings. Note the two ends of the horizontal strand are quite far apart and go over the ends of the headboard.

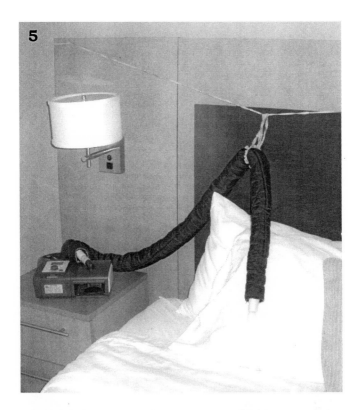

#5 – Motel A. Close up demonstrates use of the headboard when there are no pictures on the wall.

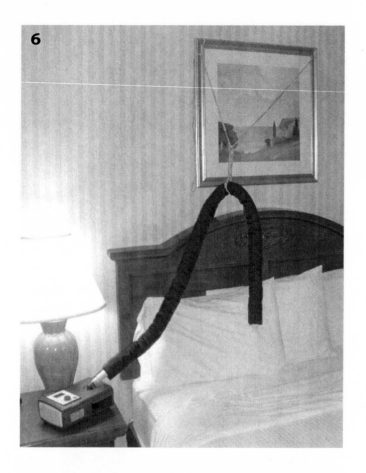

#6 – Motel B with a headboard and framed picture. Headboards can be used as in Motel A, but here the board is too low so the framed picture is used for the horizontal strand.

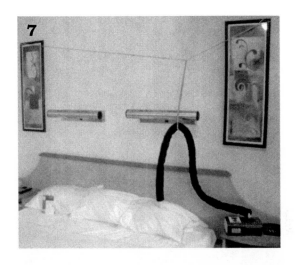

#7 – Motel C, with no picture above the bed, two wall hangings can be used.
#8 – Alternatively, the wall hangings are not used and the vertical strand is hung from the light fixture.

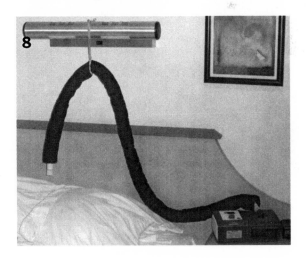

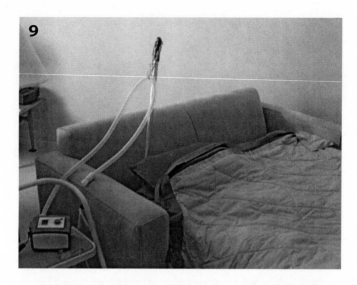

#9 – Using rubber bands to hang tube down from above when a wall or ceiling can not be used. Here the (sofa) bed was in the middle of the room. An extendable handle for a window washing attachment was used to hang the rubber bands from.

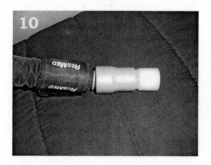

#10 – Coupler makes attaching the mask to the tube so easy it can be done with one hand.

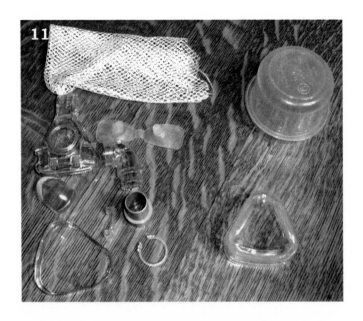

#11 – Nine mask pieces unpacked.
#12 - Nine mask pieces packed. Note the nine plastic mask pieces and the containers in which they are packed when I travel.

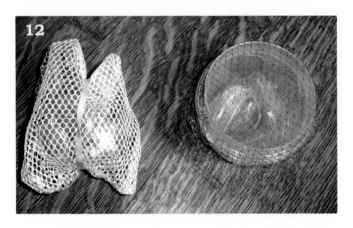

ABOUT THE AUTHOR

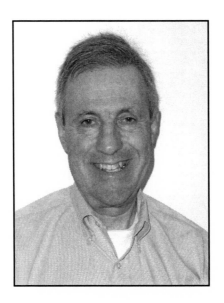

Bruce Stein was diagnosed with sleep apnea in November 1999. With the exception of about five nights, he has used a BiPAP machine every night for the past 11 years. Bruce is a pharmacist, has a PhD in biochemistry, and is an attorney who practices patent law. He used his training and experience in medical and scientific technology, as well as the creativity involved in inventions, to develop better ways to use CPAP/BiPAP.

INDEX

Note: The italic letters *n* and *p* following a page number indicate that the subject information of the heading is within a note or photo, respectively. Double italics indicate multiple but consecutive elements.

I
Infections
  airways, and humidity, 25–26
  colds as, 13
Insurance policies
  recordkeeping and, 67–68
  sleep apnea equipment in, 18, 23–24
Internet suppliers
  specific, not given, xix, 9n3
  tube coverings from, 62
Inverters, power, 43
Irritability, associated with sleep apnea, xxv
Isopropyl alcohol, as tube cleansing agent, 23
Ivory® soap, as mask cleansing agent, 21

L
Lebowitz, Fran, quoted on quality of sleep, xxx

M
Machine for CPAP/BiPAP, xiii
  attaching other parts to, 15–16, 26
  code names for, 61–62
  fuses and age of, 17–18, 33, 34
  learning to use, 38–39
  manufacturer's directions for, xxi–xxii, 29, 42
  noise of, 1, 63–65, 69–70
  power supply for, 41–43
  proper positioning of, xv, 7
  travel preparedness and, 40–41, 59
Malone, Jena, quoted on quality of sleep, xxvii, xxviii
Manufacturers
  BiPAP system directions from, xxi–xxii, 21, 22
  deviations from, directions, xix, 24
  humidifiers and their, 26
Mask for CPAP/BiPAP, 68
  assembly of, 21–22, 57–58
  attaching other parts to, xix, 15–16, 58
  booklet on, 3–4
  customary care of, 4, 22, 39, 57–58